Working Out At Home

You Don't Need a Gym Membership to Get Fit

Ron Kness

Published by:

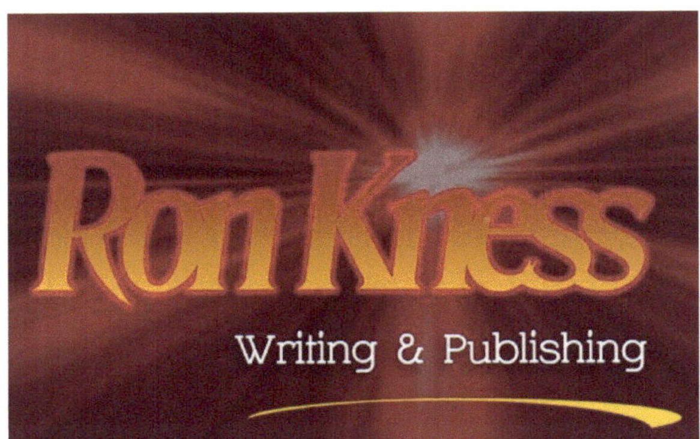

https://ronknesswriting.com
Ron Kness
Queen Creek, AZ
United States of America
For
Healthy Lifestyle Newsletter
https://healthylifestylenewsletter.com

ISBN: 9798500083678

Disclaimer

This publication is for informational purposes only and is not intended as medical advice. Medical advice should always be obtained from a qualified medical professional for any health conditions or symptoms associated with them.

Every possible effort has been made in preparing and researching this material. We make no warranties with respect to the accuracy, applicability of its contents or any omissions.

See your healthcare professional before starting any diet, health or exercise program!

Table of Contents

Disclaimer..3

Introduction 5

Time To Take Inventory 7

Cardio Exercise At Home 9

    Start Small - Go For A Walk 9

Daily Walking Workouts To Get Back in Shape 11

The Benefits Of Having A Walking or Running Buddy 13

Keep It Fun With Workout Videos..15

Weight Bearing Exercises At Home 17

    Strength Training Without Fancy Equipment 18

Create Your Own Workout Routine 20

    Workout While The Kids Play 21

Optional: Equipment To Keep An Eye Out For 23

    Using A Pedometer To Move More 24

Have You Tried A Couch To 5K App? 26

Don't Workout – Play! 28

Working In Workouts - Make It Fit Your Schedule..30

Conclusion 32

Suggested Resource..33

About the Author..34

Introduction

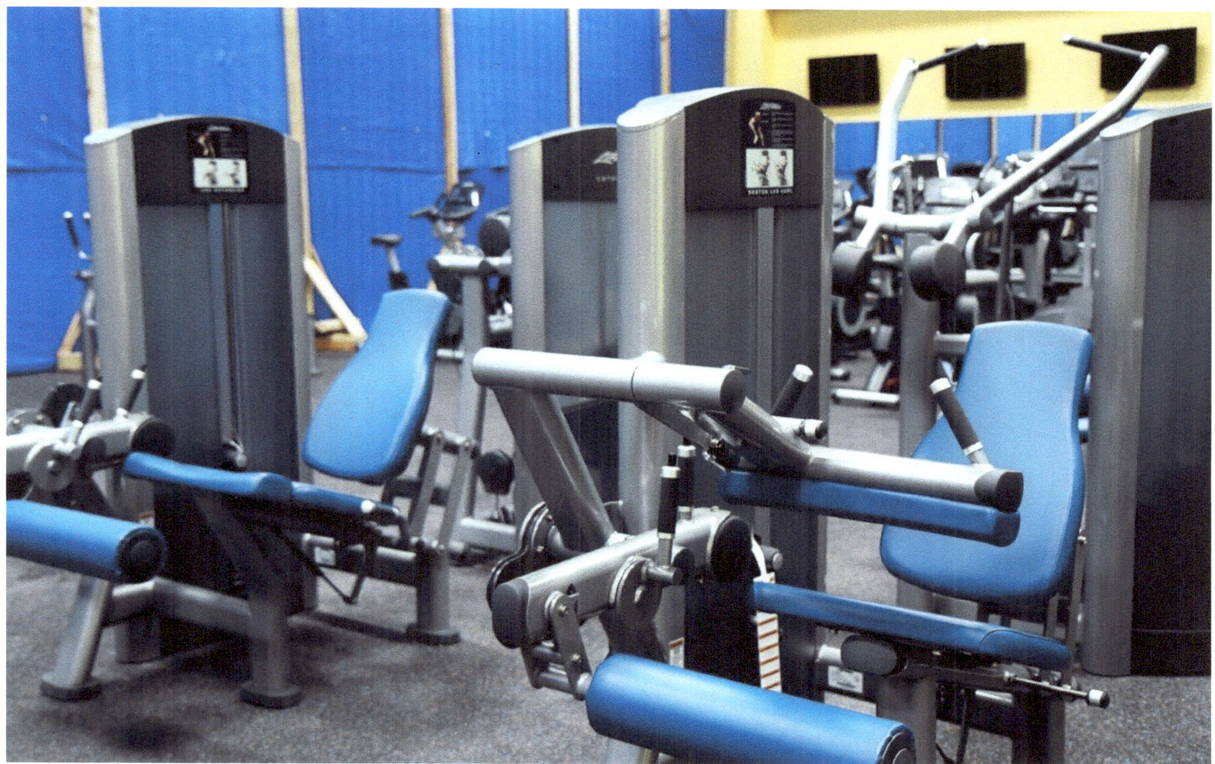

I don't have to tell you that it's important to work out and move more. Many of us live a sedentary lifestyle and drive everywhere. Our bodies weren't designed to go from sitting at the desk in our office to slumping down on the couch the minute we get home from work. We were designed to walk for miles, and work with our hands to gather food. While that isn't our daily life anymore, we do need to make an effort to work out to keep our bodies healthy and strong.

That's why there's a gym on every corner and most apartment complexes and hotels have workout rooms. Heck, there are even plenty of corporations that either have gyms onsite or work out a local deal for their employees.

But here's the thing, gyms don't work out for everyone (no pun intended). They can be expensive if you don't happen to have one in your apartment complex or are lucky enough to have a gym at your work place. And they are a time commitment. You have to get changed, drive over there, do your workout, drive back, shower etc.

Even if you keep it short, you're easily talking about a two-hour time commitment per time. And if you have a job and a family to take care of, that can be a serious challenge taking away time from your loved ones. Who has two extra hours to spend three to five times a week?

That's what makes working out at home so attractive. You can squeeze in a workout anytime you have a few minutes. You don't have to do everything all at once either.

For example, go for a walk on your lunch break and then come home and do a few sit-ups and crunches during commercial breaks while you're watching TV. You get the idea.

In this book, we'll go over some simple ways to make it easy to work out at home. You can get a great cardio and strength training workout without ever leaving your house (unless you want to).

Time To Take Inventory

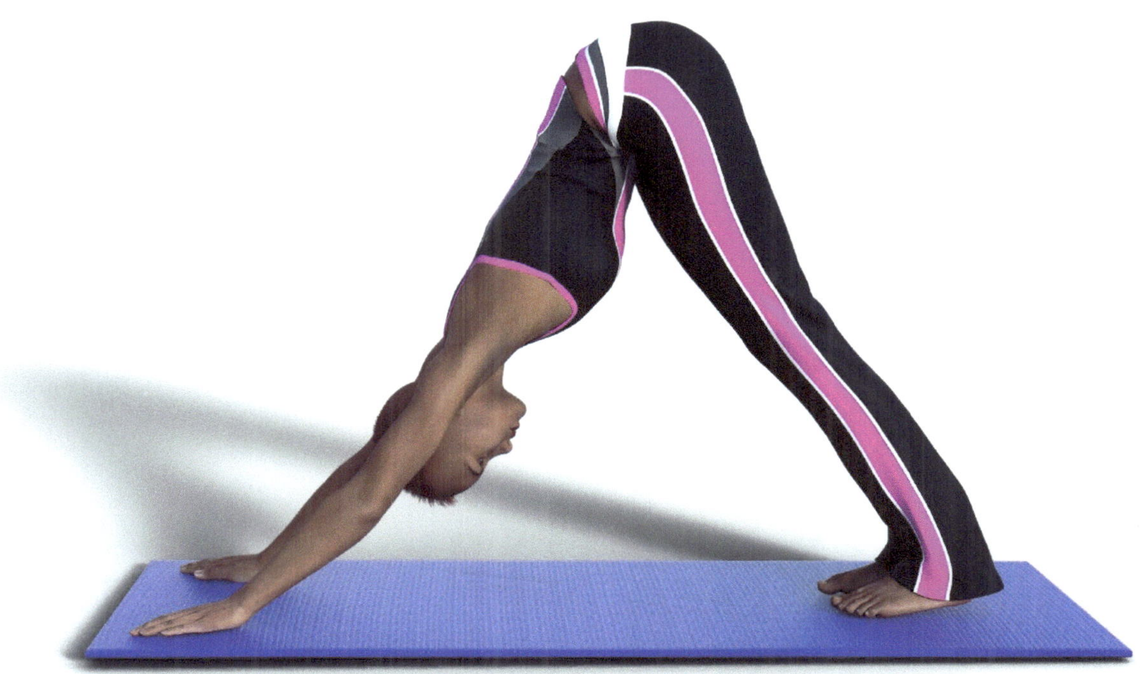

The first thing you want to do is take a good look around your house and garden, and see what you can use to work out. You'll be surprised how much you'll find once you really start looking.

Space
You don't need a lot of space to work out, but it helps if you can find an area that's large enough to give you some space to move around. A comfortable surface like carpet or a yoga mat also helps when you're stretching or doing push-ups, crunches or anything else that will have you on the floor. Your bedroom or living room are likely your best bet here.

Weights
Next, it's time to look at what you can use as weights. Canned goods work, as will small water bottles. If you need something a little heavier, try filling gallon bottles with water. Water is roughly 8 pounds per gallon.

The Furniture
Let's not forget about your furniture. Chairs, tables and counters make excellent workout equipment. You can do arm dips on chairs and counter tops. Chairs and tables also make great surfaces for elevated push-ups.

And for a real arm and chest workout, start out in front of your coffee table, put your legs on it and start doing push ups.

Old Workout Equipment and Videos
Chances are you already have some workout equipment at home. Maybe it's a stepper, an exercise bike or a treadmill that's collecting dust in the garage. Maybe it's some workout DVDs. Maybe it's a jump rope, stretch bands and a few light weights. See what you have and figure out how to use it in your new workout routine.

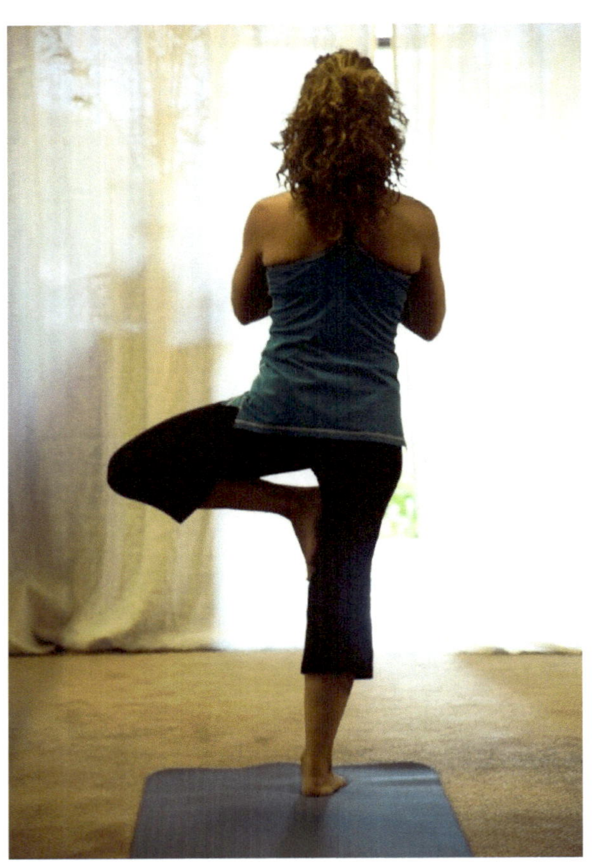

Cardio Exercise At Home

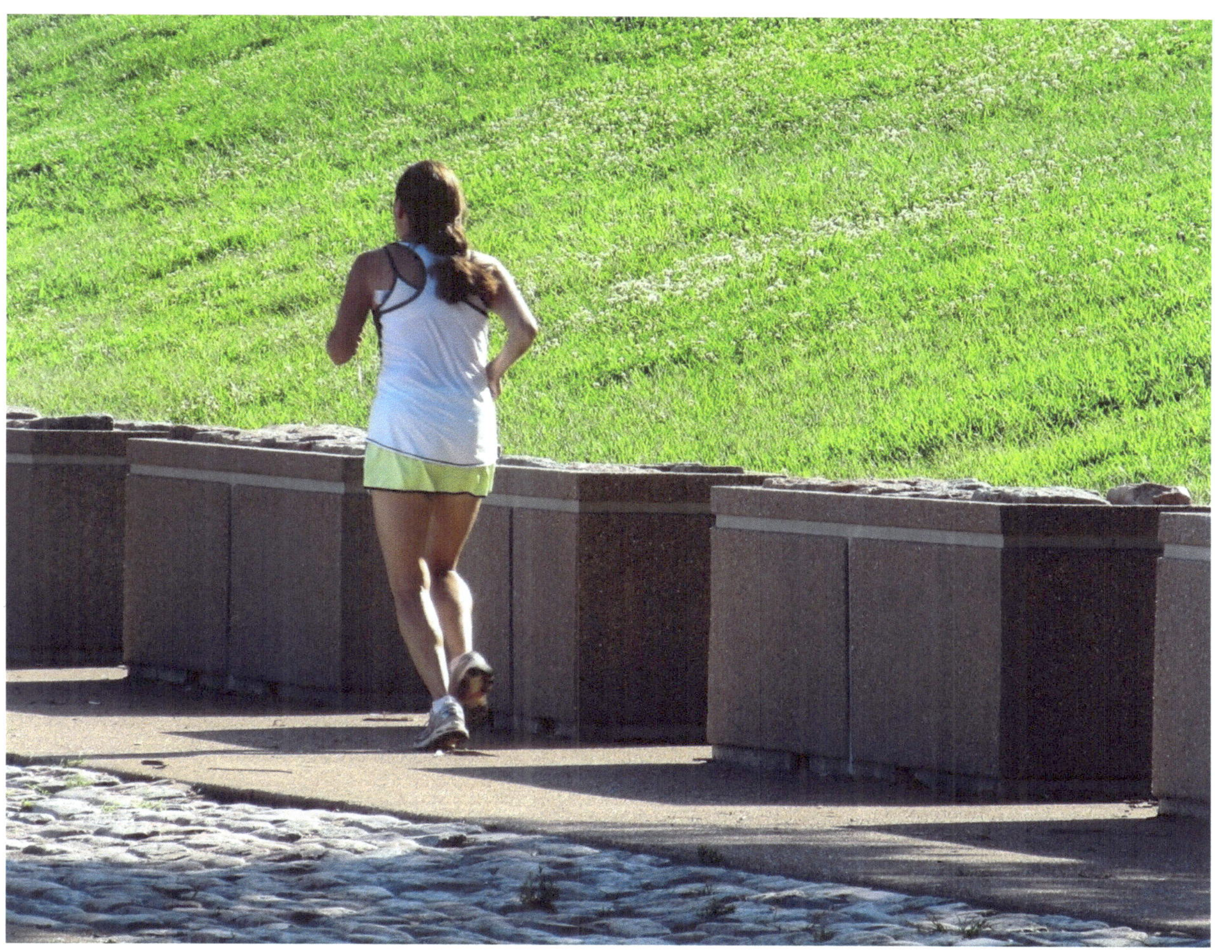

Let's start with some cardio. If you don't mind leaving the house, go for a brisk walk or a run a few times per week. All you need is a pair of sneakers and 30 to 45 minutes and you're done.

Start Small - Go For A Walk

You don't need a lot of fancy equipment to start getting in shape, particularly if you're just starting out. One of the best ways to get started is simply to walk. For that, all you need is a pair of comfortable shoes or sneakers. Let's look at what makes it the perfect way to get started, how to stay motivated to walk and how to make sure your walking workouts are effective. By the time you're done reading you'll be ready to head outside for a walk unless, of course, it's raining. Then you can put on some music with a good beat and walk around your house or walk in place.

Benefits Of Walking
Walking is a simple workout almost anyone can do. It's low impact and you don't need a lot of fancy equipment or special training to do it. It's just a matter of putting one foot in front of the other. It can be as easy or as challenging as you want it to be.

If you're just starting out, and you're not in very good shape, just take a stroll around the block each night after dinner. After a few weeks you'll be up to longer walks, picking up the pace, or tackling a small hill.

Walking gets you moving and it's a great way to get in some cardio and get the blood moving without a lot of stress on your body. At the same time, you'll start to notice that your leg muscles start to tone up and your core strengthens. It's not unusual to find that your pants are fitting looser after a few weeks of regular walks.

How To Stay Motivated To Walk Every Day
While walking is easy to do, it can also get a bit boring. If you're struggling to stay motivated to go on that daily walk, I have some tips for you...

Find a walking buddy. It's much harder to skip that walk if you know someone is waiting for you and relying on you to go with them. Having someone to talk to on your walks also keeps things interesting.

Grab your phone or mp3 player and some headphones. Listen to your favorite music while you walk, download some podcasts or lose yourself in an audiobook. Having something to listen to will make the time go by faster and keep your walks interesting and fun.

Schedule your walks and make them part of your daily routine. It will take a little while before it becomes a habit – 21 to 30 days - but before you know it you won't forget to go for your walk, just like you won't forget to brush your teeth.

Step It Up And Track What You Do
In the beginning your main goal will be to just go out there and move around. That's great and the perfect way to start out. But you'll get to a point where that quick 15-minute evening stroll isn't enough to get you the results you want. It's time to push a little harder and make sure you get stronger with each walking workout.

Start keeping track of how long and how far you walk. Set a goal each week, to either walk a bit further, or cover the same distance in a shorter amount of time.

Set a goal and then give yourself a week (or longer if needed) to get used to the new distance or speed. Once it starts to feel comfortable, you know it's time to raise the bar. Keep pushing yourself and you'll continue to get in very effective, low impact workouts by doing nothing more than walking.

Daily Walking Workouts To Get Back in Shape

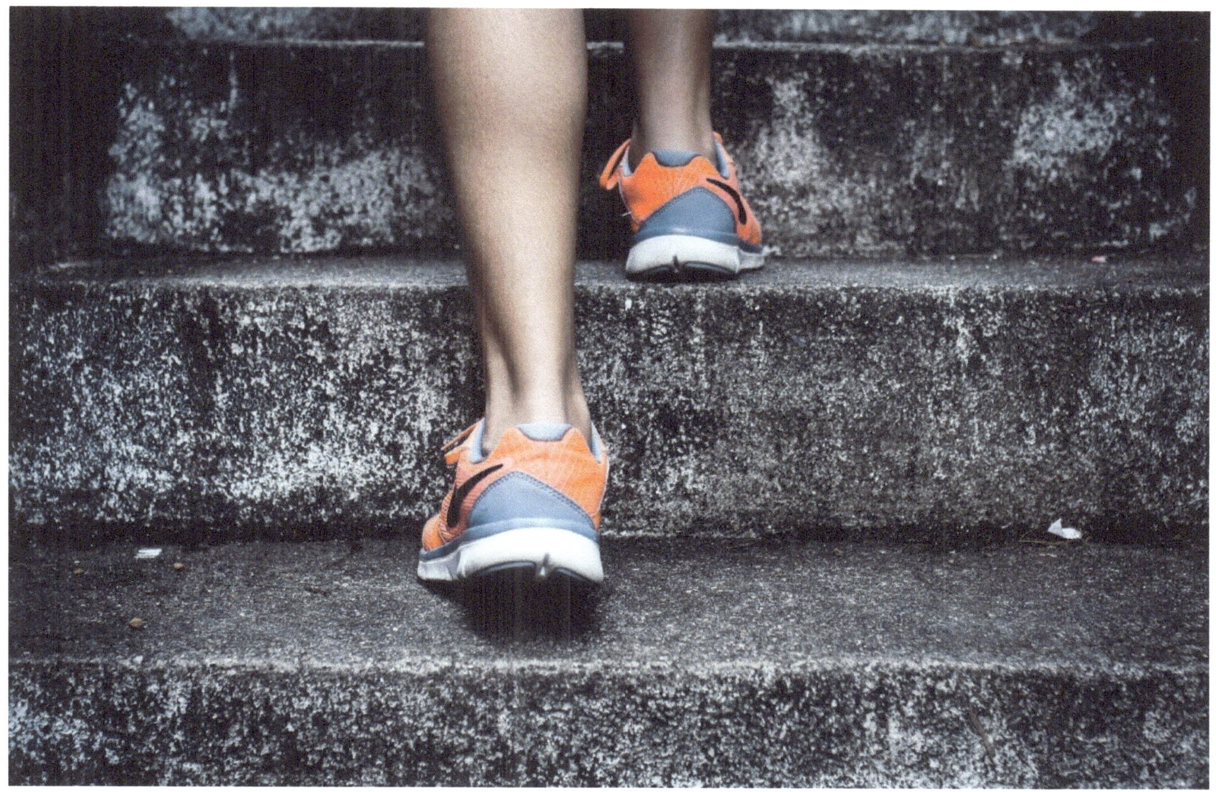

Are you ready to get back in shape? Or maybe you want to work out and improve your health for the first time. In either scenario, walking workouts are a great choice. They are easy to do. All you need to do is lace up your sneakers and head outside.

Start Small And Step It Up in 15 Minute Intervals

Any exercise is better than no exercise. Start small and do what you can for the first week or two. Put on your shoes, grab your sweater and go for a walk. If you can walk for 15 minutes, great. If you don't that's ok too. Take it slow and work your way up to 15 minutes of brisk walking. A brisk walk is defined as being able to carry on a conversation while walking.

If you can start out with a 30-minute walk at a nice steady walk, great. Start where you're at and keep it up for a week. After that time, you'll notice that your daily walk is starting to get a little easier. That's when you want to go a little further. Start increasing your walking time by 15 minutes until you get to 45-to-60-minute walks per day.

Pick Up The Pace

Eventually you'll get comfortable with your hour-long walking workouts and it's time to push a little. Start picking up the pace.

Try doing your regular walking route in less time. Keep pushing until you can comfortably do your 60-minute walk in 45 minutes. You'll start walking faster and get your heart rate up a bit.

Of course, walking further in the same amount of time is another option. Aim for a 60-minute walk but go further than you used to. Either way, the goal is to push your body a little harder to get it into better and better shape.

Work On Your Posture and Add Some Weights

Walking is a great low impact way of getting your cardio in for the week. This is particularly true once you start to pick up the pace and push yourself. But it can also be a great way to tone your body.

Start by paying attention to your posture. Keep your shoulders back and stay upright. Suck in your stomach while you walk. Not only is it a good core workout, it will also help prevent back pain from prolonged walking. As an added benefit, it will shrink your belly even faster than walking by itself.

To tone your arms and upper body, consider carrying some light weights during your walks. Two small water bottles work great. Use them to do simple arm raises or curls, or just carry them around to tone your arms and shoulders.

Take Your Walking Workouts To The Max With Interval Training

Let's wrap this up by talking about interval training. It's a great way to burn a lot of calories and push yourself to the next level. Interval training means you alternate between working out at a moderate level for a few minutes followed by 30 seconds or so of high intensity workouts and then dropping back to the moderate level again.

Start by walking at a moderate pace for 5 minutes to warm up. Then alternate 2 to 5 minutes of walking at that pace with 30 seconds to a minute of walking as fast as you can. Keep cycling through, changing the speed of your walk until you are almost back home. Slow it down a bit more to give your body a chance to cool down.

After a while, you may want to start running during the high intensity intervals. In addition to giving you a more intense walking workout, this is also a great way to transition from walking to running.

The Benefits Of Having A Walking or Running Buddy

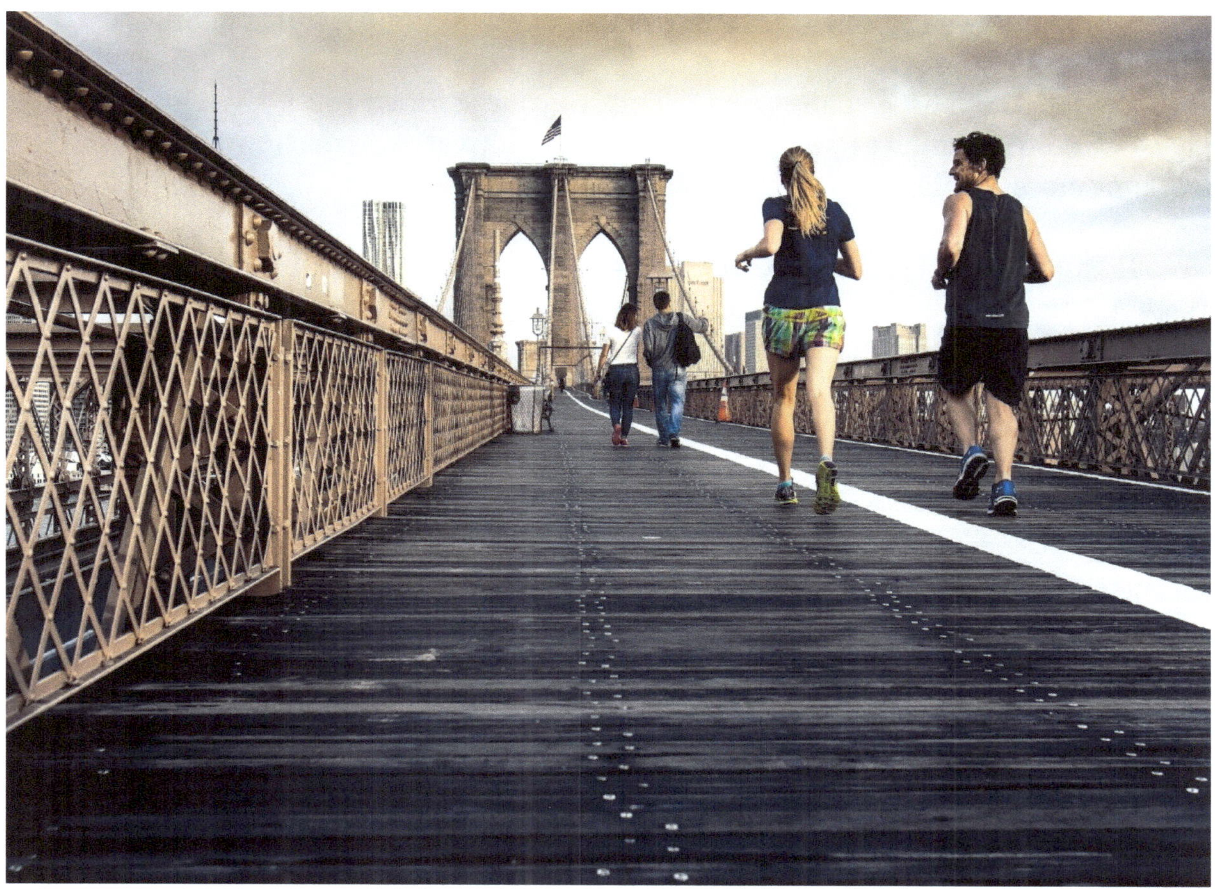

Do you have someone that goes for walks or runs with your regularly? If not, that's something you want to investigate. Having a walking or running buddy is a great way to make sure you get out there and get through your workout. Let's look at how this can help you in a little more detail.

Hopefully, it will inspire you to go find someone to hit the trails with you on a regular basis. Having someone to walk or run with you even just once or twice a week can make a big difference in how often you go work out and how much you enjoy it.

It Makes Your Workouts More Fun

Having someone to walk or run with you makes the workouts a lot more fun. And guess what? When we're having fun, we're more likely to stick with it in the long run.

You'll find yourself looking forward to chatting while you're moving along. Having someone to walk with you and talk to also makes the time go by faster. Time to find that perfect person to spend some quality workout time with each week.

You're Accountable To Your Partner
With a running buddy, you have the responsibility to show up. You don't want to let him or her down. That alone may be enough to get you out there when you're just not feeling like it. In addition, you'll encourage each other and call each other out when the other one is trying to slack off. The built-in accountability is one of the biggest benefits of having a walking or running partner and building it into a habit.

If you've found it a little challenging to stick to your workout routine week after week, give a workout partner a try and see if it doesn't motivate you to show up and workout more regularly.

You'll Push Each Other To Get Better
While the accountability is wonderful in itself, there's another powerful reason to walk or run with someone else. When we're by ourselves, we tend to set a pace that's comfortable for us. We don't often push ourselves to go faster or further. A workout buddy will do that for you. You will find you'll push each other to go a little faster and a little further.

Sometimes your walking partner will move a little faster forcing you to speed things up and sometimes it will be the other way around. Either way the end result is the same. You're both getting stronger faster and are becoming better walkers and runners.

Of course, you don't have to limit yourself to just one workout buddy. Join a walking or running group of you can find one in your area or start your own. The benefit is that you'll have people to walk or run with even when one person can't make it. The downside is that logistics get a little more complicated when you have several people and their individual schedules to consider.

If heading outside isn't an option, there's plenty you can do inside to get your heart pumping. Got a treadmill or exercise bike? Set it up in front of the TV and workout while you're catching up on your favourite TV show. You could also jump rope, walk in place or alternate doing knee lifts and jumping jacks to get in your cardio workout.

And let's not forget about workout videos.

There are plenty of routines from Zumba to kickboxing that will get you going. Invest in a couple of cardio DVDs or look around on Netflix and Amazon prime. You'll even find some fun 80s jazzercise on there. Or how about some cardio yoga and Pilates?

Keep It Fun With Workout Videos

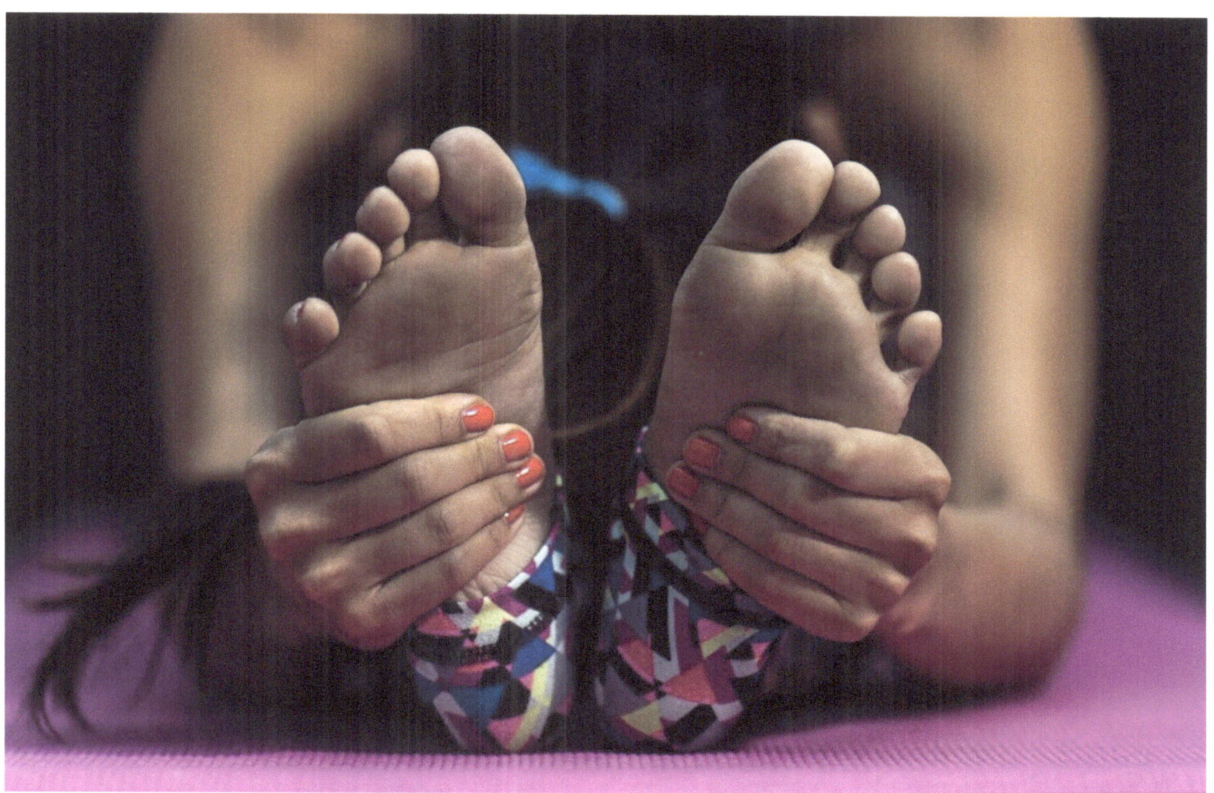

Working out from home doesn't mean you're limited to go walk or run. You can mix it up and keep things fresh and fun with workout videos. This works great on days when it's pouring down rain outside or you can't head out for your daily walk because the kids are napping or it's too dark by the time you make it home from work.

Picking different workouts is also good for your body. It keeps your muscles from getting too used to a particular routine and different ways of working out will work different areas of your body. It's good to keep your body on its toes by switching how you stay active. And let's be honest here, sometimes you just want to mix things up for the fun of it.

If you have an Amazon Prime or Netflix account take a look at the workout videos you can stream from both services. You can quite a few different workouts from kickboxing and yoga to belly dancing and Zumba. Try a few of them and see what you like. There are even some old 80's videos that will get you laughing while you're working out (ever heard of Jazzercise?)

Do a search on YouTube. You can find a variety of workouts there and if there's a particular type of instructor you like, you can look up and buy any fitness DVDs they may have. It's a nice way to test the waters and see what you like.

Did you know that you can check out videos and DVDs at the library? Check with your friends to see what they have available. Check out thrift stores and yard sales.

The idea is to borrow something or buy at a very low cost and see how you like the workout. If it's a good fit and something you can see yourself doing often, go ahead and buy the DVD.

Once you have a small collection of workout videos, mix it up and rotate through them. If you prefer more of a schedule, set them up like you would exercise classes at the YMCA. Do your Zumba workout on Monday, Walk Away The Pounds on Wednesday and get sweaty with some Tae Bo on Friday.

The key is to keep it fun and mix things up. Not only will different workout DVDs give you a better overall workout since you'll be working different muscle groups in different ways, it also keeps it interesting and most importantly keeps you from fudging your way through the routines. Keeping it fresh makes sure you stay engaged and giving it your all.

There is no excuse for not getting it done. If nothing else, crank up some music and start dancing around the house with the kids. It's a fun way to get the whole family moving.

Weight Bearing Exercises At Home

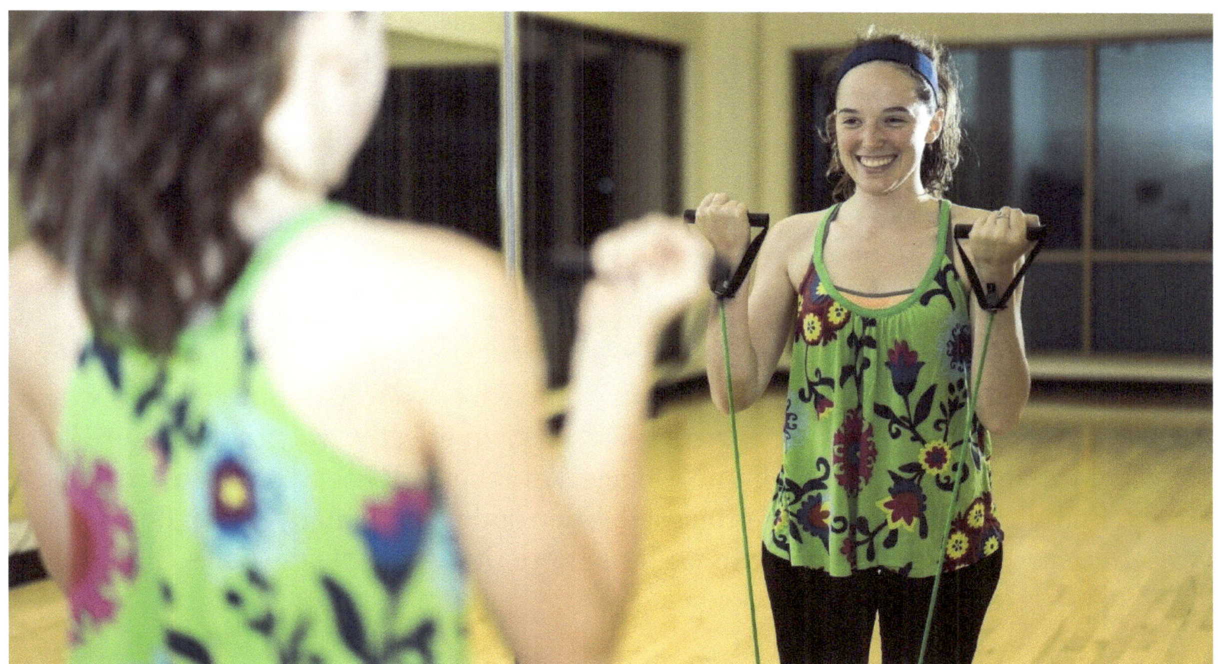

Now that the cardio is out of the way, let's talk about weights. There are plenty of benefits to doing weight bearing exercises. They include increasing your lean muscle mass which will help you burn more fat and increasing your bone density. Plenty of good reasons to include them in your weekly workout routine – something we'll talk about next.

Use cans and water bottles the same way you would hand-held weights at the gym. Or carry them as you work through your cardio workout to make it more effective.

And let's not forget about your own body weight. Push-ups, squats, and lunges are all great ways to work on those muscles. As are those chair or countertop arm dips we talked about earlier.

You can work your abs with a whole routine of different crunches and sit-ups, and you don't need anything more than a comfortable spot in the floor.

If you need a little extra challenge, grab your baby or toddler and hold her as you move through your workout routine. It's a fun way to bond and spend time with your little one while also getting a great core workout.

Look into Pilates workout videos for another great way to strengthen and tone your whole body. The exercises may look simple, but I can tell you from experience that they will make your muscles burn and are an effective way to get into shape – without any fancy equipment.

To really step it up, grab a milk crate (or a stool or chair that can hold your weight) and two milk containers (one gallon each) that you cleaned and filled with water for your workout. Step slowly up and down the crate or chair while doing bicep curls with your gallon bottles. Stabilize using your core muscles and you'll get a full-body workout with just one exercise.

Do lunges and squads the same way, switching up the arm workout routines to work different muscle groups and you'll have a workout on par with anything the gym has to offer.

Strength Training Without Fancy Equipment

You know strength training is good for you. It increases your lean muscle mass which in turn helps you burn more muscle mass. It's also an effective way to make sure your bones stay dense and strong well into old age. And that will keep you from breaking a hip or shoulder many years down the road. The good news is that you can do some very effective strength training with nothing more than a couple of chairs and cans of green beans. Here's how.

Use Your Own Body Weight

The best place to start is with your own body weight. Push ups will work your upper body and shoulder. Lunges, squats, and leg lifts will help get your legs and butt in shape. Come up with a quick and simple routine that uses nothing but your own body weight.

Chairs, Counters And Couches Make Great Tools

Look around and use what you have. Grab a chair and use it along with your body weight to work the backs of your arms and shoulders with arm dips. Use the chair for elevated push ups and give your legs another great workout by stepping on the chair and off. A quick google search for "chair workouts" will give you plenty of other ideas and detailed instructions for each workout.

For a slightly different angle and thus a workout that works different muscles, try doing the arm dips and push ups using your kitchen or bathroom counter. And let's not forget about the couch. It's a great partner when it comes to doing crunches. Stick your feet under the couch when you don't have a workout partner to hold them for you as you move through your ab workout.

Grab Those Canned Goods and Water Bottles

Working out at home without fancy equipment doesn't mean you can't lift weights and go through your regular upper body workout routine. Just head to your kitchen and grab a couple of cans of corn or green beans. Water bottles will also work well and if you need something even heavier grab to gallon water bottles at the store (or fill two empty and cleaned milk bottles with water).

They make great weights to work your arms and shoulders. Of course, the workouts will also work your core as you stabilize your body. Don't discount the relatively low weight of these containers - particularly the cans and small water bottles. They can be just as effective and make your muscles burn by doing more reps of each set of exercises.

By using what you have and thinking a little outside the box, you can get a very effective workout at home without the need to invest in a bunch of fitness equipment.

Create Your Own Workout Routine

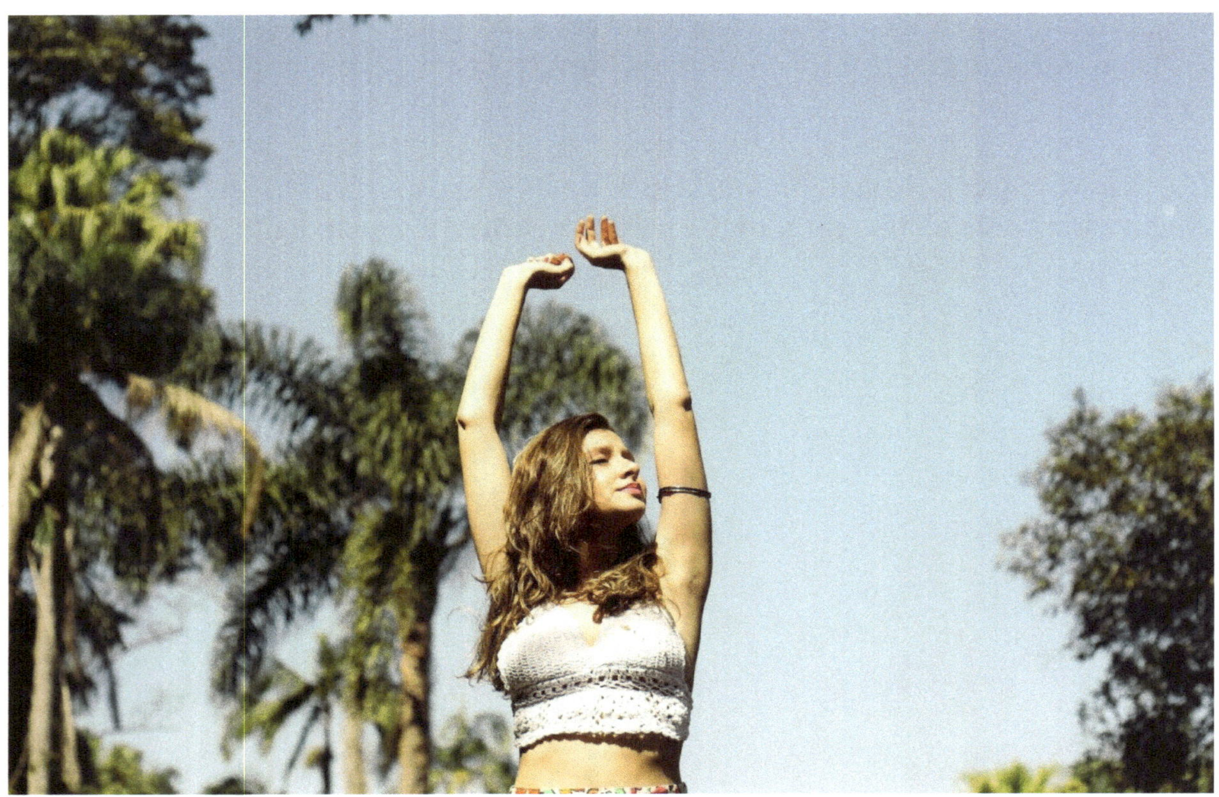

Now that we've talked about a few different ideas for both cardio and weight bearing exercises it's time for you to create your very own workout routine. Grab a pen and paper and let's get started.

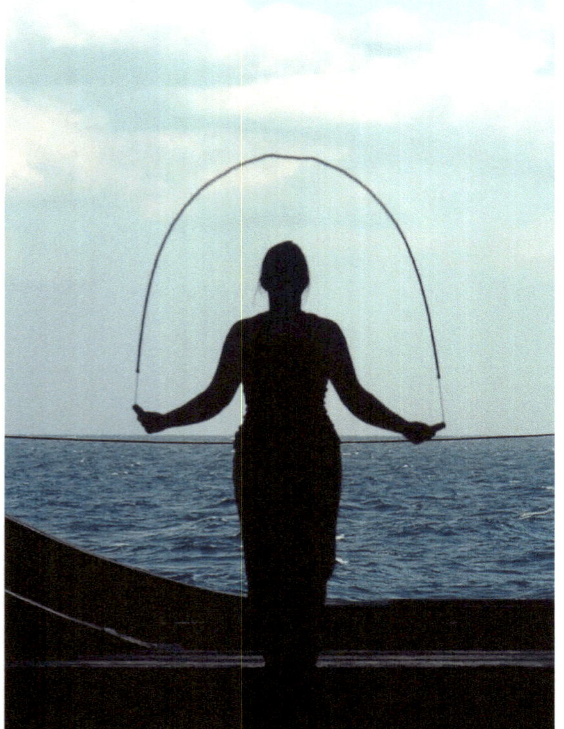

As you work through this next step make sure you know what you're doing. You need to be able to perform each exercise in a manner that's safe and effective. Google is your friend. As is YouTube.

Do your research and make sure you know what you're doing. If not, ask a friend who's familiar with workouts or even better a certified personal trainer to show you how it's done. You can pick up from there once you have your routine down.

Depending on your personal fitness levels and your goals, you may want to alternate days when you do cardio and days when you work with weights.

Or particularly if you are trying to lose weight, you may want to get in cardio every day, but also work in 3 days of weight bearing exercises.

In either scenario, make sure you give your body a day or two per week to rest. While you can still go for a walk on those day, skip the run or the jump rope workout.

When it comes to muscle building exercises, you need to give them time to recover and strengthen. That's why rotating through different muscle groups throughout the week works so well. For example, you could schedule in arm workouts on Monday, work on your abs on Wednesday and wrap up the week with leg workouts on Friday.

Figure out your routine and come up with a basic set of reps for your weight bearing exercises and some guidelines for your cardio workout. For example, you could start with a two mile walk or a one mile run.

Revise your workout plan every couple of weeks and switch things up. Try different exercises to work your body in a slightly different way. Increase the length of your cardio workout or increase the intensity by walking or running faster. Or give interval training a try. A combination of walking and running or slow jogs combined with short sprints can be a very effective way to strengthen your heart and burn a bunch of calories at the same time.

Keep your old workout routine logs. It can be very inspiring to go back and see how far you've come from when you got started. Staying motivated to work out isn't always easy. Use what you've got to stick with it and stay on track.

Workout While The Kids Play

As a parent it can be tough to find the time to work out and stay in shape. Between work, keeping the house in order and taking care of the kids there's barely enough time sleep, let alone head to the gym several times a week.

But that doesn't mean you can't sneak in a little workout here and there. The key is to multitask and do a few exercises while the kids are playing, or napping, or working out right along with you. How you make this work will of course depend on the age of your kids and your own circumstances, but here are some ideas to get you thinking.

Invest in a baby jogger if your kids are small enough to ride in a stroller. Strap them in when it's time for a nap and walk or run around the neighborhood while they sleep. If you have older kids, have them ride a bike or scooter and come along with you.

Check out the parks and playgrounds in your area. If you're lucky you can find one with a playground area in the middle and a walking path going around it. You can run or walk laps while the kids play on the playground.

And speaking of playgrounds or even the swing set you may have in your own backyard. Take a look at it and see what kind of exercises you can do on it. You may be able to find a bar that allows you to do pull ups and chin ups while the kids play. Or use the steps leading up to the playground equipment to do some simple step workouts. Get creative and make it work.

And let's not forget about just going out and playing with the kids. Go on family bike rides or take a Frisbee out to the park. Playing catch is a great way to get in an interval workout. You'll be surprised how much of workout you can get just from running around with the kiddos.

Here's one last idea for you. Get the kids involved and do your workouts together. That could mean holding your baby while you do crunches and squats. Or maybe you turn on a fun Zumba workout and have the kids dance around in the living room along with you. It's a great way to spend quality time as a family and get everyone moving around more.

Optional: Equipment To Keep An Eye Out For

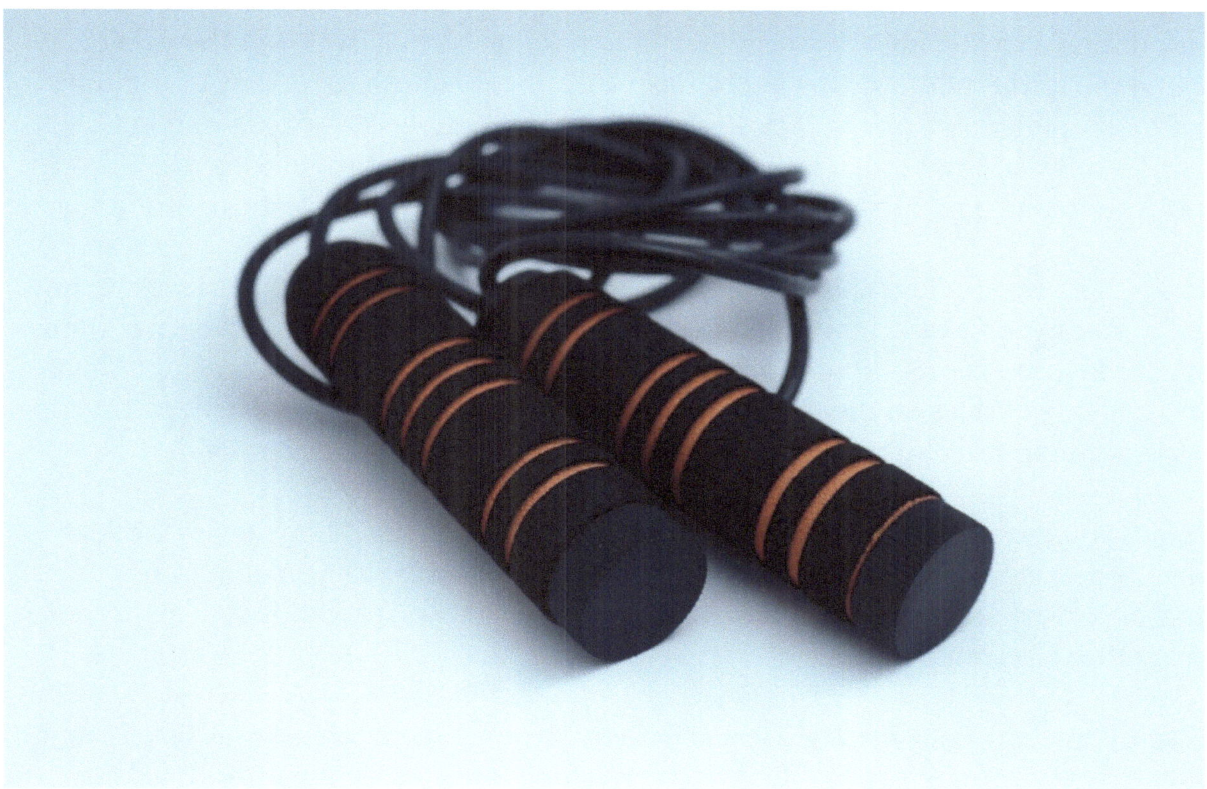

While you can get some very effective workouts in with nothing more than a couple of cans and a chair, there is also something to be said for some actual workout equipment. While this is entirely optional, it's something you may want to keep an eye out for. Find it on sale, get it used or even better see if you can get it free from a family member or friend who's no longer using it.

Jump Rope
This should be a no-brainer. Head to your favorite sports store and pick up a jump rope. It's a great cardio workout and it doesn't take up hardly any room. It's also a great portable piece of exercise equipment you can take with you when you travel.

Pedometer
If your goal is to move more and sneak your workouts in when you can throughout the day, consider getting a pedometer. You can buy something fancy like a FitBit® or go simple with a low entry level that you can pick up new for under 10 bucks.

And check your smart phone before you head to the store. Many of them have a pedometer built in and an app will help you keep track of how you're doing.

Using A Pedometer To Move More

Most of us live a very sedentary lifestyle. We get up in the morning, grab our coffee and sit down at the table. We get ready for work and sit in a car to get there. We spend the next 8 hours sitting at our desk only to get home and sit down for dinner before we plop down on the couch to watch some TV. In other words, we don't usually move around much over the course of our day. What we need is a little motivation and a way to track exactly how much (or how little) we move around.

The perfect way to do this is to use a pedometer. A pedometer will keep track of how many steps you've taken throughout the day. You can order one online or pick it up at your favorite sports supply store and clip it to your pants. You'll also find quite a few tracking devices on the market like a Fitbit® or other fitness and activity tracking devices. Some will clip to your pants or bra, others you'll wear like a watch.

Before you go out and buy a device, check your smart phone. Many newer models have pedometers built in. If you carry your phone around with you at all times, it may be a great way to track your steps and your activity level without having to invest in another electronic device.

Start by tracking your normal level of activity. Just go about your day as usual and note how many daily steps you take. Track it for a week and come up with a daily average. Write that number down. Chances are it will be well below the recommended 10,000 steps per day. For some of it will be quite a bit less than half that number. That's ok. It's just a starting point.

Your next goal is to increase your average by 1,000 steps per day. Start parking a little further away from your office, walk over to ask a colleague a question instead of calling and go for a short walk after dinner.

Keep tracking your daily steps and increase your daily goal by 1,000 steps every few weeks until you make it a habit to walk at least 10,000 steps. It's not as hard as you may think and the beauty of doing this instead of a walking workout or a daily trip to the gym to hop on the stationary bike or treadmill is that you can get more active in little spurts throughout the day. Walk around while you are talking on the phone, park in a central location and walk from store to store as you shop, take a quick stroll on your lunch break.

You'll find all sorts of different ways to sneak in a little more activity throughout your day. Before you know it, you'll reach and surpass your 10,000-step goal and won't be able to imagine moving around less.

Treadmill

A treadmill is a great way to get your walk or run in when the weather is bad, or you're tied to the house because the kids are sleeping. New they are expensive but they are also big sellers so chances are good that you can pick one up used. Start asking around and see if someone in your family or your circle of friends has one they are no longer using. Craigslist is another good place to look.

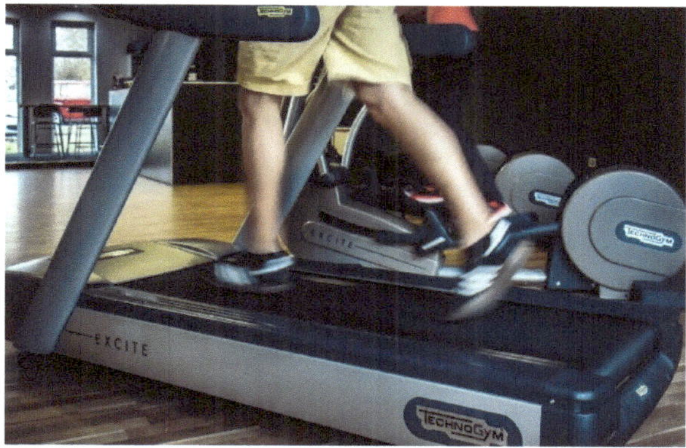

Stationary Bike

The same goes with stationary bikes. If you are having a hard time walking or running, a bike might be a better option. While they don't seem to be quite as popular as they have been in the past, you should be able to find a used model. Set it up in front of the TV or bring your laptop and watch a movie or TV show while you cycle away.

Free Weights

While canned goods work great, and gallon water bottles give you more weight to work with, you will reach a point where you need more flexibility or heavier weights. Keep an eye out for a set of free weights. Look for a set with removable plates so you can adjust and change as needed.

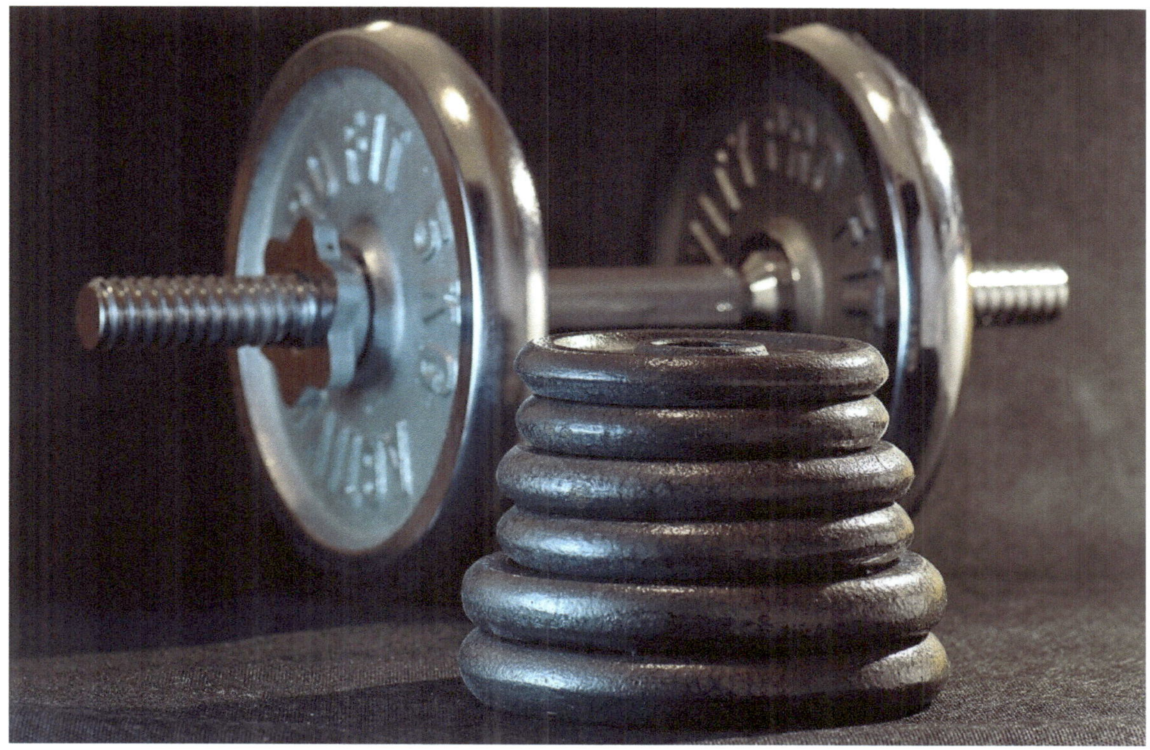

Have You Tried A Couch To 5K App?

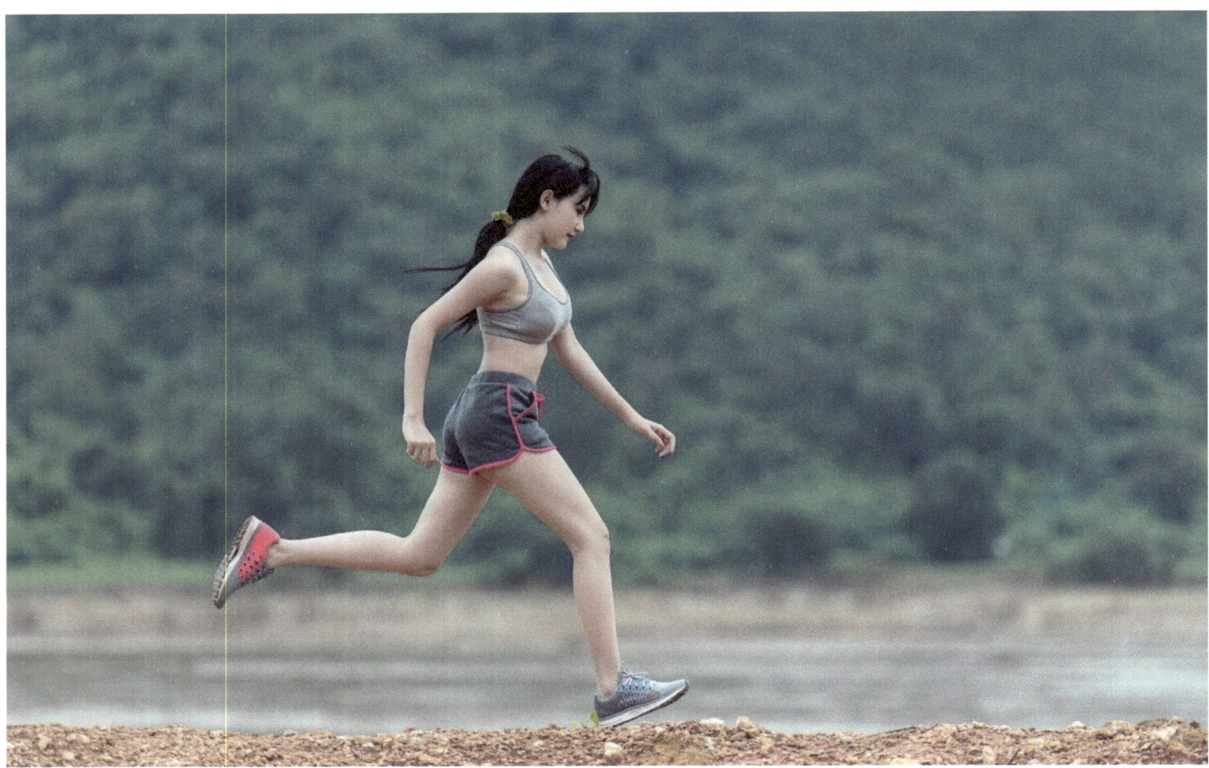

Running is a great overall workout that you can do anywhere and a wonderful way to make sure your body and your heart stay in great shape. But if you're a bit of a couch potato, going out for a run can seem a bit challenging.

Not to mention that you'll be out of breath after 2 minutes. As easy as running is, if you're out of shape, it isn't something you can pick up and do for long – at least in the beginning. Let's just say you won't be going for a 5K run on your first day. But it's something you can work up to in a few short weeks.

There are plenty of Couch to 5K programs out there. You can find books on the topic, blogs and email courses. The basic concept is the same. These programs lead you through a mixture of walking and running exercises for a few weeks until you are ready to run your first 5K.

It's a great way to get in shape and while the books, blogs and ecourses certainly work, one of the best ways to do a couch to 5K is with a phone app. Yes, you read that right. Your smartphone can be a great tool to get you moving and then running.

The way these apps work is that you run it while you're walking and running with headphones on. Your phone will tell you when to walk, when to run and when to do other exercises as you move through your daily workouts.

While you'll get a lot of the same information and go through the same exercises and steps with a book or other way to go through the couch to 5K program, there are some very specific benefits to using an app.

Typically, you will walk for a few minutes, and then run for a minute and so forth. If you're working with written information you must remember what you're supposed to be doing and then time yourself. The app will keep track of all that for you and tell you what to do each step of the way.

The app will also keep track of what day and what particular workout you're on. It makes it easy to know where you're at in the program, but it also has a motivational aspect to it. Seeing on your screen that you've already completed 2 weeks' worth of workouts can be very motivating.

Last but not least, most apps will remind you that it's time to do your workout. That may be just the little nudge you need to lace up your sneakers and go work out.

Don't Workout — Play!

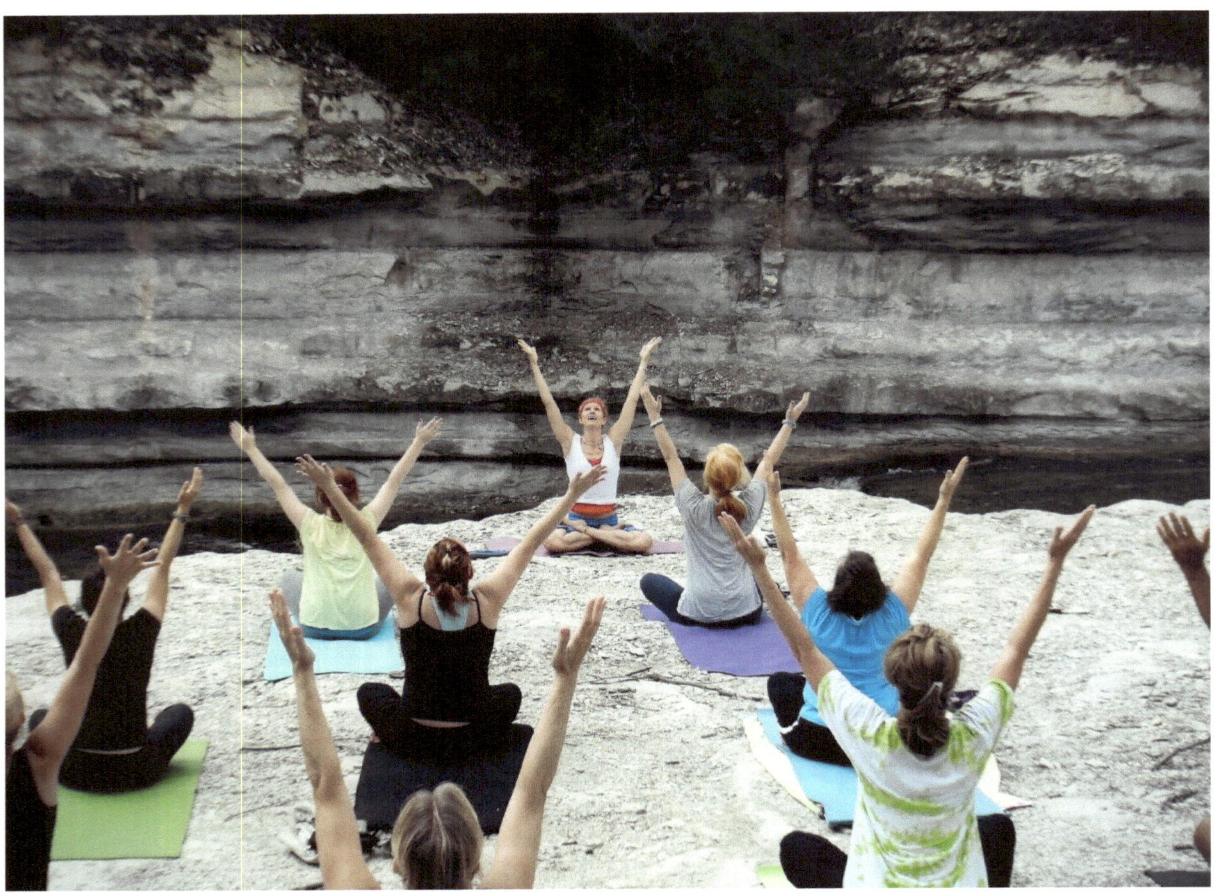

If you're dreading to have to go get your workout in every day, then don't. No, I'm not suggestion you give up on getting or staying in shape and turning into a couch potato. What I am suggesting is that you change things up and stop thinking of it as working out. Instead, think of it as playing. And playing to stay in shape can take many different forms.

Make Walking Fun
If you're getting tired of your daily walk, consider taking someone along with you. It's a nice way to break up the routine and have someone to talk to while you walk.

Another good option is to download an audiobook or your favorite podcasts and listen to them while you walk. It will make the time go by much faster and you'll do something else you enjoy while you walk.

Join A Team Sport
There's a reason they call it playing a team sport. Think about what you like to do and find a team around there. Think baseball, softball, volleyball and the likes. Or how about tennis or golf? Join a bowling league or give pickle ball a try.

Not only will you get a great workout, you'll also get to hang out with a fun group of people that love to play and make working out a lot more enjoyable.

Try A Few Workout Classes
If you're a member of a gym or the "Y", consider taking a few different workout classes. The goal is again to find something you enjoy that feels more like playing than working out. Who knows, it could be the yoga class you haven't tried, or maybe you find your love for belly dancing.

If you don't want to join a gym, rent a few different workout videos and see what's fun. Once you have that figured out, you can either stick with the workout DVDs, or look for a local class that's similar.

Go For A Hike Or A Bike Ride
The weekends are the perfect time to take your workouts to the great outdoors. Get the family together and go for a hike or a long bike ride. You can fit a whole lot of working out into one of these outings and spend quality time with your loved ones at the same time. Of course, the added benefit is beautiful scenery and plenty of sunshine and fresh air.

Splash Around In The Water
Let's not forget about playing in the water. Who doesn't like to splash around? Look for a local pool, a lake or if you're lucky enough to live close to the beach head out for a swim in the ocean. Swimming itself is a great low impact workout, but it doesn't stop there. Check out the water aerobics classes at your local pool and see if that's a fun way for you to get in your cardio and strength training.

Working In Workouts - Make It Fit Your Schedule

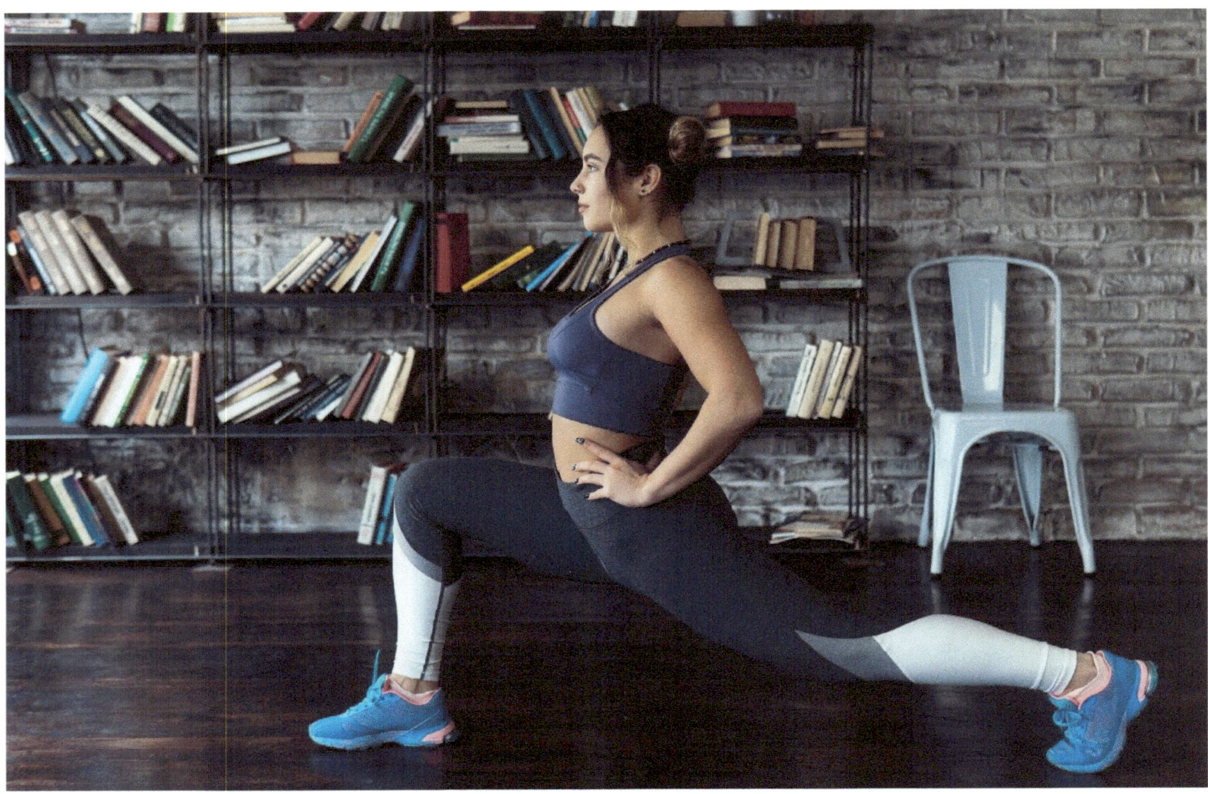

Here's an important concept when it comes to working out. If you're waiting for there to be time in your busy schedule, it's never going to happen - at least not on a regular basis. You must make working out a priority and part of your daily or weekly schedule. But that doesn't mean you have to drop everything else.

The first important thing to realize is that there is no right or wrong way to exercise. If getting up 45 minutes early so you can go for a run before work works for you, great. But if it doesn't, don't fret it. That run will be just as effective late in the afternoon after work, or even at night on the treadmill.

You also don't have to do everything in one block of time. Working out in five- or ten-minute intervals can be just as effective. Research has proven that three 10-minute workouts are just as effective a one 30-minute one. As a matter of fact, the three are more effective because each time your metabolism increases and stays increased for several hours afterward. With one 30-minute workout, your metabolism increases only once.; with three workouts, it increases three times and one increase could carry over to the next. Burn more calories and lose more weight.

Do a few stretches when you first get up in the morning and do your sit-ups during commercial breaks while you're watching TV at night. By fitting workouts in here and there throughout the day, you can get a lot done without having to rework your entire schedule.

Of course, it helps if you can block out some dedicated time to work out. But if you're busy, that may take some creative thinking. Getting up early so you can get your workout in before the rest of your day takes over is of course an option. But it isn't the only one. Schedule a quick workout and a packed lunch at your desk during your lunch break. Go for a walk or head to the gym next door while you're waiting for your kid at piano lessons. Look through your schedule and find those little pockets of time that would otherwise be wasted. Instead of sitting in your car for 30 minutes to wait on your child, get out and move around.

Last but not least, I want you to realize that it's ok to take the time to go work out. Making sure you're in shape and are doing something for yourself makes you a much better parent, spouse and friend. It's not selfish to schedule in a workout three days a week or head out for a run after work.

Take that time to make sure you stay in shape. Not only will you feel better if you do, chances are you'll avoid a slew of health issues down the road that would otherwise take you away from your family and loved ones for much longer than the few hours per week you spend working out.

Conclusion

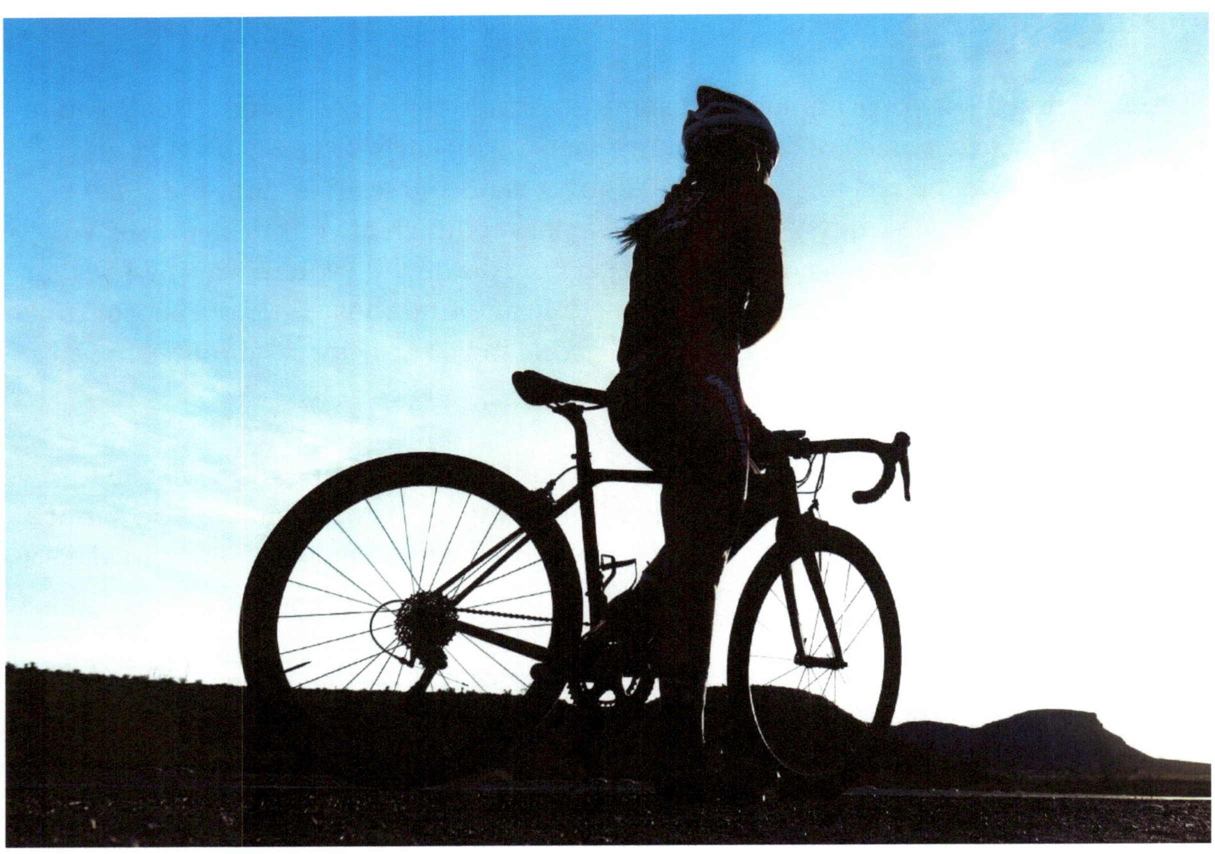

Working out isn't always easy, but making it as convenient as possible – by working out at home – can be a big help. The key is to get started and stick with it for a few weeks. You'll be pleasantly surprised how quickly you will start to see results. You'll feel better, look better and sleep better.

Come up with your workout routine and stick with it until it becomes a habit. Yes, there will be days when you won't feel like working out. It happens to all of us. The trick is to get started. Tell yourself you only need to do one set of arm exercises, or walk down to the end of the road and back. Once you get moving it gets easier and before you know it you will have gone through your entire routine.

Give it a try and get moving. It's well worth the effort.

Suggested Resource

If you are interested in learning more about exercising, get my new book" Getting *Healthy: 5 Permanent Lifestyle Changes That Help Achieve Your Fitness Goals*".

In it, you will learn how to make small changes in your daily life that add up to big benefits when it comes to achieving your fitness goals. But, I hate to break it to you, but there is no easy way to get healthy, lose weight or get back into shape. It takes time and it takes dedication.

Yes, it would be nice to have a magical pill or an easy button. That's the reason there's such a huge market for diet pills and weight loss gimmicks. But the hard truth is that they just don't work.

What works is making lifestyle changes and sticking to them. That's what this book is all about. I'm not promising that it will be easy as pie or that you'll lose 50 pounds overnight.

What I can promise is some helpful information that will allow you to make those lifestyle changes. I'll show you how to create good habits that will help you reach your goals. After that it's up to you to implement them and finally get healthy – for life.

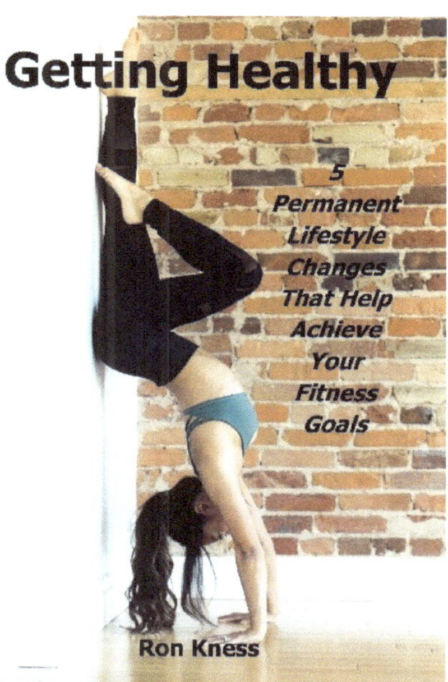

Are you ready to get started getting healthy?

Get your copy at: https://www.amazon.com/dp/B093Z5RNXH

About the Author

I am a published writer with numerous books on Amazon for Kindle and other publishing platforms ... both in electronic and Print On Demand (POD) formats. While most of my self-published books are on health and fitness in general, my topics

 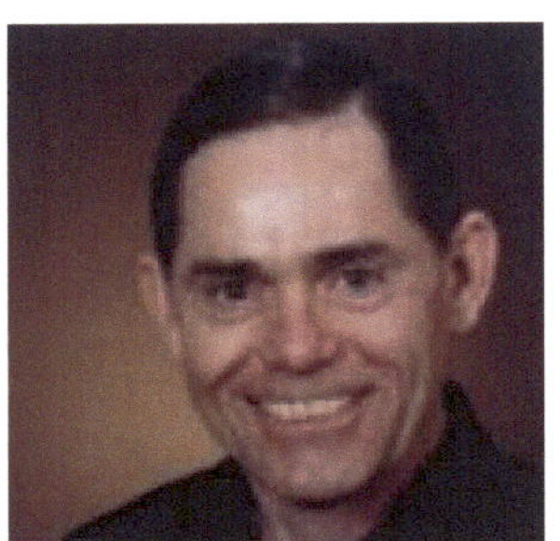

of interest currently are more toward 1) aging baby boomers and the older population and 2) low content books, like word activity books, journals, planners and calendars.

Besides my own writing, I also ghostwrite ebooks, books, reports, articles, autoresponder series, blogs and Kindle conversions for my client base on a variety of topics. I'm currently using Microsoft's Office Suite including Word, Powerpoint and Publisher, along with Affinity Publisher and Designrr for writing and publishing.

Go to my website at http://ronknesswriting.com for more information or to request a quote: https://ronknesswriting.com/ghostwriting-quote-request-form.

For a complete list of my books published on Amazon, go to https://www.amazon.com/Ron-Kness/e/B0072M6PYO..

Today my wife and I are retired from our careers and live in Queen Creek, AZ. I now write as a retirement business where you'll find me happily sitting in my office typing away on my computer as I work on my next book or ghostwriting project for a client . . . that is if we are not traveling somewhere in our RV - our renewed mode of travel.

Take care and be safe!

Ron